Optivia Diet Cookbook

Over 40 Lean & Green

101+ Easy and Healthy Optivia Diet Recipes or Beginners and Advanced Users to Burn Fat and Get Lean Achieve Rapid Weight Loss For a Healthy

By   KATY SMITH

© Copyright 2022 - All rights reserved.

Disclaimer Notice:

Please note the information contained within this document is for educational and entertainment purposes only. All effort has been executed to present accurate, up to date, and reliable, complete information. No warranties of any kind are declared or implied.

Readers acknowledge that the author is not engaging in the rendering of legal, financial, medical or professional advice. The content within this book has been derived from various sources.

Please consult a licensed professional before attempting any techniques outlined in this book.

By reading this document, the reader agrees that under no circumstances is the author responsible for any losses, direct or indirect, which are incurred as a result of the use of information contained within this document, including, but not limited to, errors, omissions, or inaccuracies.

TABLE OF CONTENT

Introduction

The term OPTAVIA may seem unfamiliar; it's actually an increasingly popular weight loss plan that severely restricts calories and recommends eating a mix of branded processed foods called fuels and homemade lean and green meals.

The word "Optavia" might sound like a new prescription drug or even a brand of eyeglasses, but it's an incredibly common weight loss strategy that's gaining momentum online. In its year-end survey, Google listed Optavia as one of the top diets in 2018, and Cake Boss star Buddy Valastro also credited his recent drastic weight loss to the program.

"A lot of people have asked me how I've been losing weight recently, so I felt the need to share that I used the Optavia app," he posted last June on Instagram. "I'm not paying to say it, and it must be remembered that I believe everyone is unique and you can do something that suits you, so that's what I'm doing, and I'm very happy with the results so far!"

Officially nothing is off limits, especially on a diet, so it's not just a walk with pies. The software severely restricts carbs and is urging its members to get "supplies" to lose pounds.

"In general, it's hard to suggest strict diet plans like Optavia," says Jaclyn London, head of nutrition at the Good Housekeeping Institute. "While transparency and support are the main components of any behavior improvement plan, behavior therapy with unhealthy eating practices causes many of us to have disordered eating behaviors and limit - binges - limited impulses."

At least half of every Optavia diet consists of its "supplies," including chips, drinks, cakes, pasta, and some savory choices, such as broth and mashed potatoes. These packaged foods also mention the first ingredient as whey protein or soy protein. Lean, nutritious foods take up most of the diet you buy and cook yourself.

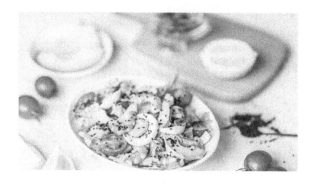

CHAPTER 1:

Basics of the Optavia diet

What is the Optavia diet

The Optavia diet concept was introduced by the team behind Medifast, a popular meal replacement company. Following the Optavia program requires eating low-calorie, low-carbohydrate foods. You will need a combination of packaged foods and homemade meals to effectively lose weight. If you don't like cooking or are the busy type and don't have enough time to cook your meals, the Optavia diet will be great for you as it doesn't require you to cook for long.

• It is important to note that while Medifast does not require individual coaching, the Optavia diet does.

- The Optavia diet improves weight loss through branded products known as refueling, while homemade appetizers are referred to as lean and green meals. The supplies consist of over 60 items that are specifically low in carbohydrates but are high in probiotic cultures and protein. The supplies also contain friendly bacteria that can help improve gut health. They include; biscuits, bars, puddings, smoothies, soups, cereals and pasta.

- Looking at the foods listed, you might think they are quite high in carbohydrates, which is understandable, but the supplies are compounded in such a way that they have less sugar and carbohydrates than traditional versions of similar foods. The company does this by using small portions and sugar substitutes. Additionally, many of the fuels are high in soy protein isolate and whey protein powder. Those who are interested in the Optavia diet, but are not interested in or do not have the ability to cook, are given prepackaged low-carb meals from the company. These meals are referred to as Flavors of Home and can sufficiently replace lean and green meals.

- The company explicitly states that by working with its team of coaches and following the Optavia diet as required, you will achieve a "permanent transformation, one healthy habit at a time".

- Therefore, to register success with this diet program, you need to stick to foods that are supplemented by vegetables, meat and healthy fat appetizer every day - you will be full and fed. Although you will consume few calories, you will not lose a lot of muscle as you will feed on lots of fiber, protein and other vital nutrients. Your adult calories will not exceed 800-1,000. You can lose 12 pounds in 12 weeks if you follow the optimal weight plan option 5 and 1.

- Since you will reduce your carbohydrate intake during this diet, you will naturally lose fat because carbohydrate is the main source of energy, so if it is not readily available, the body finds a fat alternative, which implies that the body you have to break down fat to get energy and keep burning fat.

- The Optavia diet is an idea from Medifast and includes pre-purchased snacks and portioned meals, low-carb (homemade) lean and green meals, and ongoing coaching based on facilitating fat and weight loss.

• Optavia is a weight reduction or maintenance strategy that prescribes consuming a combination of refined and imported meals - called "refueling" - and "healthy and fresh" prepared meals. There are no sugars and calories to log. Followers often apply water to dried food or unpack a bar as part of six or more small meals a day. Optavia also provides instructor advice to help you understand copyrighted "Fitness Habits".

• However, the package recommends doing about 30 minutes of moderately intense training each day.

• The Optavia diet is a diet rich in proteins, including proteins that provide 10-35% of the calories per day. But the dried and powdered kind can have some less than pleasant results.

• "The protein extract with additives will make people bloated or have some unpleasant GI side effects that will make you feel better in a sugar-free Greek protein yogurt smoothie," London says.

• Additionally, the FDA does not check the protection and effectiveness of dietary supplements like smoothies and powders as it does with food. "Protein powders and 'blends' can contain unhealthy additives or interfere with a drug you may be taking," says London, "making it especially important to make sure your doctor understands you're on the diet."

• To promote weight reduction, Optavia relies on intense calorie restriction. Both "supplies" are around 100-110 calories each, which ensures you are consuming only 1,000 calories per day on this diet.

• London believes there is a healthier solution to sustainable weight loss: "Eat meals and snacks that contain lots of vegetables, 100% whole grains, almonds, beans, legumes and legumes, low-fat dairy, meat, fish and lean beef with few indulgences is the perfect way to sustainably lose weight in the long term. "

• There is also some reduction in carbohydrates behind the scenes. Since carbohydrates are the primary source of energy, limiting them leads the body to the best substitute fuel available: fat. OPTAVIA is advised to cut down on carbohydrates just enough to start losing fat - you will consume 80 to 100 grams per day.

• Medifast Inc. is the parent organization of Optavia. It still runs and maintains the Medifast service you can call back from the 1980s and 1990s, which used to see doctors recommending meals to their patients. Optavia provides common foods with an equivalent macronutrient profile, so customers should sign up directly for the package.

Possible benefits of the Optavia diet

• The Optavia diet has many benefits that can be achieved when practiced according to its "strict" guidelines. Some of the advantages are:

•

• **It is easy to follow**

• Taking the diet is very simple as it is mostly based on prepackaged supplies and all 6 meals you will need to take per day, whereas with the 5 & 1 plan, you will only have to cook 1 of the meals.

- For each plan you decide to take, you will be provided with a sample meal plan and meal logs that will help you maintain your diet.

- You can only cook a maximum of 1-3 lean, green meals per day based on the type of schedule you are on and these meals are simple to prepare. You will be given a list of specific food options and recipes that you can always choose from.

- The programs can also help improve patients' blood pressure through weight loss and a low sodium intake. Optavia meals are well prepared, providing less than 2,300 mg of sodium per day, which is the U.S. Department of Agriculture (USDA) recommended daily sodium intake level.

- **Helps to lose weight**

- The diet contributes / helps people who actively wish to lose weight and excess fat. It does this by reducing the number of calories and carbohydrates consumed through its well-controlled portions and snacks. Studies have shown that a reduction in overall calorie intake can lead to more significant weight loss; this is when complete or partial meal replacement habits accompany it.

- **The coaches offer their support**

- Health coaches involved in the Optavia diet are often available for advice during the weight loss or weight maintenance journey. And research has shown that having access to a lifestyle coach can help maintain weight over time.

- **Ability to improve blood pressure**

- The Optavia diet program can improve participants' blood pressure as there will be low sodium consumption and weight loss.

- **Ongoing support**

- Once enrolled in the Optavia program, you will have access to the coach assigned to you for the entire cause of the programs. This applies to whichever plan you choose, whether it be for weight maintenance or loss. The numerous coaching sessions associated with the program have been shown to significantly increase weight loss among program participants.

• Low sodium intake that reduces the risk of blood pressure and heart disease, lifestyle coach support that has been effective in achieving significant weight loss and maintenance, flexibility of eating plans making it easy to follow, ability to Losing excess weight and fat in a few and many more are some of the benefits you can get by joining the Optavia diet program.

Possible Disadvantages of the Optavia Diet

• Although the Optavia diet is an effective tool for weight loss, it has some potential drawbacks. Some of its drawbacks are:

• **Low calorie consumption**

• The Optavia diet can only contain 800-1,200 calories consumed per day during the 5 & 1 plan, which is very low for an adult consuming more than 2,000 calories before then.

• While low calorie intake can significantly lead to weight loss, it can also lead to muscle loss.

• Studies have shown that low calorie diets can lead to frequent hunger and cravings, which can make it more difficult to stick to the diet plan.

• **It can be difficult to remain faithful**

• Plan 5 & 1 of the Optavia diet program includes 5 prepackaged supplies and 1 lean, green (low carb) meal only. This shows that the program has limited food options and a low calorie count; therefore, it can be difficult to maintain. Since the food options are limited and not what you are used to, you can tire down the line during the program, and as such, you can easily develop cravings for other foods and cheat the diet.

• While the maintenance plan is not as restrictive as the other 2 control plans, it also depends mainly on supplies.

• **The Optavia diet plan can be expensive**

• The Optavia diet can be expensive regardless of which plan you choose.

• An average of 3 weeks of Optavia supplies, which can be on the order of 120 servings, while on the 5 & 1 plan they can cost between $ 350- $ 450. However, this cost will also include coaching for that period, but does not cover the grocery cost for recommended lean and green meals.

- ## Why and how is the Optavia diet better than keto and other diets?

- While the keto diet often limits carbohydrate consumption significantly, much of the diet is made up of fat and some protein as well. The Keto diet was originally meant for people suffering from neuropsychosis. While the rest of the food in the Optavia diet is prepackaged, highly refined, full of chemicals and sweeteners. Yes, much of the food you consume is unhealthy, refined, and even expensive.

- If you choose to lose weight more efficiently and comfortably, Optavia will be your nutritional benchmark. But you will bear the possibility of severe food malnutrition, muscle weakness, and mental health disorders at the same time. This lifestyle could prove to be ineffective, toxic, and quite expensive for you in the long run. You may end up losing the weight you lost as it is difficult to sustain long-term value with this diet and is not as sought after.

• Is Optavia a diet containing ketogenic? No, this diet is not like the ketogenic diet, an incredibly low carb plan. You are consuming a lot of fat on a keto diet, a small amount of protein, and relatively few carbohydrates. The meal plan turns into almost no fruit consumption, hardly any grains like rice and bread, and lots of high-fat foods like avocado, beef, and olive oil.

• Optavia's software could be a good solution for you if you want a simple and easy to follow diet plan that helps you lose weight easily and includes comprehensive social support.

WhyIs the Optavia diet the best choice for weight loss?

Throughout the year, the Optavia diet created a colossal advertising campaign. This weight loss initiative allows consumers to sign up for something like a low calorie meal plan, then purchase the processed meals that are part of their preferred plan. In all of this low calorie program, which offers "permanent change, one good practice at a time", no food category is out of bounds.

Optavia isn't inexpensive, but many fans have won the food. It was rated second by the United States in the rapid weight loss group. Data and World Survey, and in 2018 it was a flagship diet on Google. Friend "Cake Boss" Valastro owes his new weight reduction to Optavia.

You must follow the Optavia diet and can it help you lose weight? Here's what you need to know: If this organized strategy is difficult to execute, the chances of keeping weight reduction at bay forever and what the health risks might be.

Optavia's low calorie existence has advantages and disadvantages. While weight reduction isn't as easy as calories introduced or calories eliminated, 1,100 calories is a substantial cut from what most of us eat on an average day, so you are likely to lose weight fast early, particularly. with the 5 & 1 diet. "You can show success early on whenever you consume a low calorie," says dietician Brittany Model, MS, RD, CDN.

To keep it at bay? The challenge awaits us. "Our bodies are really smart, over time they can compensate for the low-calorie diet by going into 'hunger' mode," says Modell. "If you lose more than two pounds a week, you can tend to use your lean body mass rather than fat." Plus, even if you plan on refueling every two hours, you'll always feel diet hungry.

Some disadvantages of Optavia include loneliness and social alienation. "I think a meal replacement diet could be a start to the weekly menu strategy, but with the monotony, it could present a problem," says Tony Castillo, a spokesperson for RSP Fitness. (Aside from that, there's no doubt it's hard to pick a cereal bar when friends hit a happy hour.)

Refueling from Optavia isn't necessarily easy either. If you follow the plan, be prepared for a financial commitment. Meal replacements range from $ 400 to $ 450 for four weeks.

An advantage of Optavia is its built-in training capability. Diet is a valuable support mechanism that can help people meet their weight reduction goals. Fuels solve the question of whether to consume and what for those looking for order. And the packaging and portability of those take-away meals promise sheer versatility for busy days.

Is this diet recommended by dieters?

While you could use Optavia to help you lose weight fast, most dieters aren't really a big fan. Castillo states that while the diet might skip weight loss, it's certainly not a long-term remedy. "In the long run, meal replacement doesn't really work, so you keep focusing on prepackaged ready-made meals and snacks. Instead, strive to find a strategy that fits your needs in the best way to get the results you expect."

According to Modell, "My biggest suggestion will be not to use food substitutes," he notes. "Even so, if you don't use them, I suggest that you bring some healthy, unrefined foods back into your diet like fruits and vegetables. Eating healthy meals is essential."

Why choose this diet to lose weight quickly and not go hungry?

Throughout the year, the Optavia diet created a colossal advertising campaign. This weight loss initiative allows consumers to sign up for something like a low calorie meal plan, then purchase the processed meals that are part of their preferred scheme. In all of this low calorie program, which offers "permanent transformation, one healthy habit at a time," no food category is out of bounds.

Although it has many fans, Optavia is not cheap. The US news and world report ranked it second in the fast weight loss category. In 2018, it was also a trending diet on Google. "Cake Boss" Buddy

Valastro owes his new weight reduction to Optavia.

• Do you want to try the Optavia diet? Will it really help you lose weight? Here's it all for you: the health implications, if it's hard to follow, and the likelihood of reaching your weight loss goal.

• Optavia's low calorie existence has advantages and disadvantages. While weight reduction isn't as easy as calories introduced or calories eliminated, 1,100 calories is a substantial cut from what most of us eat on an average day, so you're likely to lose weight fast early, particularly with the 5 & 1 diet. "You can see success early on whenever you consume low calorie," says dietitian Brittany Modell, MS, RD, CDN.

• To keep it? The challenge awaits us. "Our bodies are really smart; they can, over time, compensate for the low-calorie diet by going into "starvation" mode, "says Modell." If you lose more than 2 lbs. a week, you can tend to use your lean body mass rather than fat. "Plus, although intend to refuel every two hours, you will always feel hungry for diet.

• Some disadvantages of Optavia include loneliness and social alienation. "I think a meal replacement diet could be a start to the weekly menu strategy, but monotony can be a problem," says Tony Castillo, spokesperson for RSP Nutrition. (Aside from that, there's no doubt it's hard to pick a cereal bar when friends hit a happy hour.) Refueling at Optavia isn't necessarily easy either. If you follow the plan, be prepared for a financial commitment. Meal replacements range from $ 400 to $ 450 for 4 weeks.

• An advantage of Optavia is its built-in training capability. Diet is a valuable support mechanism that can help people meet their weight reduction goals. Fuels solve the question of whether to consume and what for those looking for order. And the packaging and portability of those take-away meals promise sheer versatility for busy days.

Is this diet recommended by dieters?

• While you could use Optavia to help you lose weight fast, most dieters aren't really a big fan. Castillo states that while the diet could aid weight loss, it is certainly not a long-term remedy. "In the long run, meal replacements don't really work, so you keep focusing on prepackaged meals and snacks. Instead, strive to find a strategy that fits your needs in the best way that you can get the results you expect. "

• According to Modell, "My biggest suggestion will be not to use food substitutes," he notes. "Even so, if you don't use them, I suggest you bring back some healthy, unrefined foods like fruits and vegetables in your diet. Eating healthy meals is essential. "

• Why and how is the Optavia diet better than keto and other diets?

• While the keto diet often limits carbohydrate consumption significantly, much of the diet is made up of fat and some protein as well. The keto diet was originally meant for people suffering from neuropsychosis. While the rest of the food in the Optavia Diet is prepackaged, highly refined, full of chemicals and sweeteners. Yes, much of the food you consume is unhealthy, refined, and even expensive.

• If you choose to lose weight more efficiently and comfortably, Optavia will be your nutritional benchmark. But you will bear the possibility of severe food malnutrition, muscle weakness, and mental health disorders at the same time. This lifestyle could prove to be ineffective, toxic, and quite expensive for you in the long run. You may end up losing the weight you lost as it is difficult to maintain long-term value on this diet if you don't study it.

• Is Optavia a diet containing ketogenic? No, this diet is not like the ketogenic diet, an incredibly low carb plan. You are consuming a lot of fat on a keto diet, a small amount of protein, and relatively few carbohydrates. The meal plan turns into almost no fruit consumption, hardly any grains like rice and bread, and lots of high-fat foods like avocado, beef, and olive oil.

Chapter 2: Optavia Foods

You have a general idea of the types of foods allowed for the Optavia diet. You will find a more defined list in this segment. Use it as a quick reference when planning your meals!

In the Optavia 5 and 1 plan, the only foods allowed are Optavia Fuelings and one lean, green meal per day.

These meals consist mostly of lean proteins, healthy fats, and low-carb vegetables with two recommended servings of fatty fish per week. Some low-carb condiments and drinks are also allowed in small amounts.

The foods allowed in the daily Lean and Green meal include:

- Meat: Chicken, turkey, lean beef, game, lamb, pork chop or tenderloin and ground beef (at least 85% lean)

- Fish and shellfish: halibut, trout, salmon, tuna, lobster, crab, shrimp or scallop

- Eggs: Whole eggs, egg whites or egg whips

- Soy products: only tofu

- Vegetable oils: rapeseed, flaxseed, walnuts and olive oil

- Other healthy fats: low-carb salad dressings, olives, low-fat margarine, almonds, walnuts, pistachios, or avocado

- Low-carb vegetables: kale, spinach, celery, cucumbers, mushrooms, kale, cauliflower, eggplant, zucchini, broccoli, peppers, spaghetti, squash, and jicama

- Sugar-free snacks: Popsicles, jelly, chewing gum and mints

- Sugar-free drinks: water, unsweetened almond milk, tea or coffee

- Condiments and toppings: dried herbs, spices, salt, lemon juice, lime juice, yellow mustard, soy sauce, salsa, sugar-free syrup, zero calorie sweeteners, just ½ teaspoon ketchup, cocktail sauce or barbecue sauce

During the transition phase and plan 3 and 3, you are especially encouraged to eat berries compared to other fruits, as they have less carbohydrates. These are just a few reasons:

They are "loaded with antioxidants that help maintain free radicals under control. Free radicals are unstable molecules that are beneficial in small amounts but can damage cells when their numbers become too high, causing oxidative stress. "

Sample menu

Here's what the Optimal Weight 5 & 1 plan might look like one day:

- Replenishment 1: Golden Chocolate Chip Essential Pancakes with 2 Tbsp (30ml) Sugar-Free Maple Syrup

- Supply 2: Essential Drizzled Berry Crisp Bar

- Supply 3: Essential Jalapeño Cheddar Poppers

- Supply 4: Essential Homemade Chicken & Vegetable Flavored Noodle Soup

- Fueling 5: Essential Strawberry Shake

- Lean green meal: 6 ounces (172 grams) of grilled chicken breast cooked with 1 teaspoon (5 ml) of olive oil, served with small amounts of avocado and salsa, plus 1.5 cups (160 grams) of vegetables mixed cooked such as peppers, courgettes and broccoli

- Optional snack: 1 fruit flavored sugar-free fruit pop

The Optavia Diet promotes weight loss through low calorie prepackaged foods, low carb homemade meals, and personalized coaching if you choose to use it.

While the initial 5 & 1 plan is quite restrictive, the 3 & 3 maintenance phase allows for more variety of foods and fewer processed snacks, which can make weight loss and long-term adherence easier. However, the diet is expensive, repetitive, and doesn't meet all dietary needs. Additionally, extensive calorie restriction can cause nutrient deficiencies and other potential health problems.

Although the program promotes short-term weight and fat loss, more research is needed to assess whether it encourages the permanent lifestyle changes necessary for long-term success.

Foods to avoid

With the exception of carbohydrates in prepackaged Optavia Fuelings, most carbohydrate-containing foods and beverages are prohibited on Plan 5 & 1. Some fats are also limited, as are all fried foods.

Foods to avoid - unless included in supplies - include:

- Refined cereals: white bread, pasta, cookies, pancakes, flour tortillas, crackers, white rice, cookies, cakes or pastries
- Fried foods: meat, fish, shellfish, vegetables and sweets such as pastries
- Some fats: butter, coconut oil, or solid fat
- Whole dairy products: milk, cheese or yogurt
- Alcohol: all varieties
- Sugary drinks: fruit juice, energy drinks, soda, sports drinks or sweet tea

The following foods are prohibited during Plan 5 and 1, but added during the 6-week transition phase and allowed during Plan 3 and 3:

- Fruit: all fresh fruit

- Fat-free or low-fat: milk, cheese or yogurt

- Whole grains: High-fiber breakfast cereals, wholemeal bread, brown rice, or wholemeal pasta

- Legumes: peas, lentils, beans or soy

- Starchy vegetables: Sweet potatoes, white potatoes, corn, or peas

Preparing the lean and green meal using an air fryer

In food plan 5 and 1, dieters are allowed one healthy homemade meal per day. Of course, in the other plans, this number is expanded, allowing dieters more opportunities to experience healthy foods at home. During the first few weeks of my program, I barely had time to unwrap a chocolate bar and sit down to lunch. When it came to making my own homemade meal, I was overwhelmed with the possibility of having to grab a cutting board and start cooking a healthy meal from scratch. After all, I craved some food already prepared for me that I could simply plate and eat. I decided to talk to my health coach about it and was surprised by his suggestion.

I decided to take his suggestion and buy my air fryer. Thankfully, I have never regretted making that investment. The air fryer is everything my health coach said it would be and more! The air fryer is a guilt-free, healthy way to make my favorite deep-fried foods that meet the Lean and Green regulations of the Optavia diet. Fried foods are cooked with circulating heat instead of the traditional method of using gallons of oil in a deep fryer. As such, air fried foods have a lower fat content than other popular fried foods. This easy-to-use kitchen gadget is useful for dieters like me who want to lose weight while also enjoying some of their favorite culinary dishes.

The air fryer offers convenience in cooking delicious meals

My air fryer can pretty much do it all. By all this I mean that it can fry, bake, roast and grill meats and vegetables. It also has the ability to cook multiple dishes at the same time by simply stacking foods on top of each other. However, this is not all. The air fryer also prepares food in minutes, reducing the time it takes to prepare and consume my meals. This gadget is the master when it comes to making healthy and affordable meals cooked in the shortest amount of time.

No more fat and no more mess

My memories of fried foods are not pleasant. I remember being afraid of the splashes of hot oil on my skin and the cumbersome cleaning I had to do on the hob and kitchen countertops next. Fortunately, with an air fryer, you don't need oil to make crispy, flavorful stir-fries. This also means that I no longer have to put up with grease stains on serving plates, fingers and kitchen countertops.

Preparing meals in an air fryer is quick and hassle-free

Air fryers are lifesaving for people like me who are always short on time. It only takes a few minutes for an air fryer to cook crispy golden fries or crispy chicken legs. I would recommend the air fryer for individuals, parents and professionals who are constantly on the go and don't have much time during the day to prepare meals. The less time spent in the kitchen ultimately translates into more time spent on other activities and activities.

CHAPTER 3:

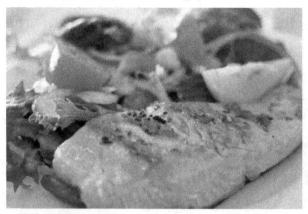

Meal plans

A deeper look at the Optavia diet

The Optavia diet encourages people to limit the number of calories they should be consuming on a daily basis. Under this program, dieters are encouraged to consume between 800 and 1000 calories per day.

For this to be possible, dieters are encouraged to opt for healthier foods and meal replacements. But unlike other types of commercial diet regimes, the Optavia diet comes in several variations. There are currently three variations of the Optavia diet plan that you can choose from according to your needs.

Diet plan 5 & 1 Optavia

This is the most common version of the Optavia diet and involves taking five prepackaged meals from Optimal Health Fuelings and a balanced homemade meal. 4 & 2 & 1 Octavia Diet Plan

This diet plan is designed for people who want to have flexibility while following this regimen. Under this program, dieters are encouraged to eat more calories and have more flexible food choices

. This means they can consume 4 Optimal Health Fuelings prepackaged foods, three home cooked meals from Lean and Green, and one snack per day.

Optavia 5 & 2 & 2 diet plan

This diet plan is perfect for people who prefer to have a flexible eating plan to achieve a healthy weight. It is recommended for a wide variety of people. In this diet regimen, dieters are required to eat 5 meals, 2 lean and green meals, and 2 healthy snacks.

Diet plan 3 and 3 Optavia

This particular diet program was created for people who have moderate weight problems and just want to maintain a healthy body. Under this diet plan, dieters are encouraged to consume 3 prepackaged optimal foods and three home cooked meals.

This plan is specially designed for weight maintenance. It consists of 3 supplies of Optavia and 3 balanced lean and green meals per day.

In addition to these 3 plans, the Optavia program improves weight maintenance and weight loss with tools such as giving inspirational tips via text messages, weekly support calls, community forums, including an app designed to set meal reminders and monitor food intake and activity.

People with gout, diabetes, nursing mothers, teens, and the elderly all have specific plans offered by the company that is designed solely based on their condition. Although specialized programs exist for people with special medical conditions, you may need to speak to your doctor if you have an individual medical condition before proceeding with the program.

Nursing mothers and teenagers also have specific daily calorie intake that may not be achieved if they follow the Optavia diet plan. Hence, it is best for anyone in this category to speak to their doctor before starting to avoid future health complications.

Opt for nursing mothers

This diet is designed for mothers who are breastfeeding with babies of at least two months. In addition to supporting nursing mothers, it also encourages gradual weight loss.

Opt for diabetes

This Optavia diet plan is designed for people who have type 1 and type 2 diabetes. Diet plans are designed so that dieters eat more green and lean meals, depending on their needs and condition.

Opt for gout

This diet includes a balance of low-purine and moderate-protein foods.

Optavia for seniors (aged 65 and over)

Designed for the elderly, this Optavia diet plan has some variations that follow the components of Fuelings depending on the needs and activities of the elderly dieticians.

Optavia for teenage boys and Optavia for teenage girls (13-18 years)

Designed for active teens, Optavia for Teens Boys and Optavia for Teens Girls provide the right nutrition for growing teens.

Regardless of the type of Optavia diet plan you choose, it's important that you speak to a trainer to help you determine which plan is right for you based on your individual goals. This is to make sure you get the most out of the plan you have chosen.

CHAPTER 4:

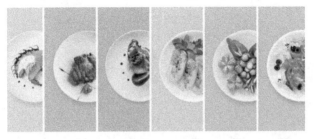

How to implement the transition period for the other phases

How easy is it to follow this diet?

When embarking on a new diet regime, you may encounter some difficulties along the way. Below are the reasons why this diet is considered the easiest to follow among all the commercial diet regimens.

Eating out can be challenging but still possible

If you like eating out, you can download the Optavia dining out guide. The guide includes tips on how to navigate buffets, order drinks, and choose toppings. In addition to following the guide, you can also ask the chef to substitute the ingredients used to cook your food. For example, you can ask the chef to serve no more than 7 ounces of steak and serve it with steamed broccoli instead of baked potatoes.

Opt for lean, green foods with a high satiety index

Eat foods that are high in protein and fiber as they can keep you full for longer periods. In fact, many nutrition experts point out the importance of satiety when it comes to weight loss.

You have access to competent coaches

If you follow the Optavia diet plan, you have access to experienced coaches and become part of a community that will give you access to support calls and community events. You also have a standby nutritional support team who can answer your questions.

Currently, the Optavia diet is ranked in the top 22 easy-to-follow diets; this is made possible mainly due to the wide range of options it offers its customers, as there are over 60 refueling options to choose from at any given time. But despite all this, you can still be tempted to walk away from the plan, but the upside is that you are allowed to eat a couple of hours during which you don't need to keep track.

In 2010, a study by Nutrition Journal described in detail in the weight loss section; found that most of Optavia and other dieters had dropped out of the program for 40 weeks. But overall, according to the Diabetes Educator study, the Optavia diet has a higher level of retention than other diets.

One of the best ways to stick to your plan is to rely on Optavia coaches and other tools and resources available online. The Optavia guide gives you ideas on the type of lean and green meals you can try; it also gives you ideas on how to modify your recipes to effectively fit the schedule.

How to start this diet

The Optavia diet consists of several phases. A certified coach will instruct you on the steps you need to take if you want to follow this regimen. But for the sake of those who are new to this diet, below are some of the things you need to know, especially when you are still getting started with this diet regimen.

Initial steps

During this phase, people are encouraged to consume 800 to 1,000 calories to help you lose at least 12 pounds within the next 12 weeks.

For example, if you're following the Optavia 5 & 1 diet plan, you need to eat 1 meal every 2 to 3 hours and include a 30-minute moderate workout most days of the week.

It is necessary to consume no more than 100 grams of carbohydrates per day during this phase.

Aside from these things, below are some other things you need to remember as you go through this step:

Make sure the recommended serving sizes are for the cooked weight and not the raw weight of the ingredients.

Choose baked, broiled, broiled or poached foods. Avoid frying foods as you will increase your calorie intake.

Eat at least two portions of fish rich in Omega-3 fatty acids. These include fish such as tuna, salmon, trout, mackerel, herring and other cold water fish.

Choose meatless alternatives like tofu and tempeh.

Transition phase

There should be a slight increase in daily calorie intake with different food groups each week. This is done in weekly stages.

Phase 1: Additional vegetables

Phase 2: Fruit

Phase 3: Dairy product

Step 4: Whole grains

CHAPTER 5:

Exercise tips

When it comes to maintaining a healthy lifestyle by losing weight, exercise is very essential. During weight loss, you need to burn more calories than you consume. Regular exercise can be so beneficial to the brain too.

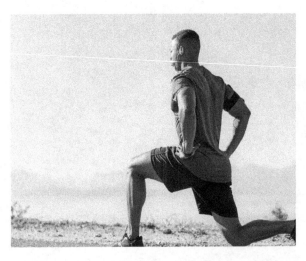

You don't have to exercise to lose weight, but it helps. If you decide to add exercise, you should do a combination of cardio and strength training. Cardio helps you burn more calories and strength training will keep your muscles. It is important to preserve muscle while losing weight because muscle burns calories. If you don't train for strength, you will likely lose muscle as you lose weight.

When you imagine someone who is fit and healthy, what does he look like? Usually, your mind may gravitate towards the image of a person who is chiseled and physically thin. Obviously that person didn't become like that just because he eats salads all day. Yes, diet is a very important aspect of fitness. There is no doubt about it. However, that's only half the story. Not all the work you do for fitness is done in the kitchen. You also have to work out in the gym.

You need to engage in proper and consistent exercise if you really want to lose weight.

Of course, in theory, you would be able to lose weight on diet alone. However, by simply sticking to diet and no exercise, you are hindering your progress. You have the opportunity to truly accelerate your progress on your weight loss journey if you are able to combine a strict diet with an effective exercise routine. So even if you're not the most athletic person in the world, you'll want to consider adopting an exercise routine for yourself.

It will be very difficult to sustain a physically active lifestyle. However, you know this is something you need to do for your own good. It's incredibly troubling these days in the age of technology that machines are starting to make people's lives easier. Yes, there is irony in that sentence. It is true that technology has made the lives of people around the world much easier and more convenient. However, it also encouraged laziness and inactivity among so many people. Why do something yourself when a machine can do it for you? Even simple household tasks like sweeping or vacuuming can be done by a robot now. There is a lot more incentive for people to sit still and relax all the time.

This is exactly why the fitness industry is more important than ever. Due to the fact that machines do most of the work that humans were responsible for, people now need an outlet to stay physically active. So, to get you on the road to getting physically fit, let's first discuss what constitutes proper training and exercise.

It can get really uncomfortable when you carry a lot of excess weight all the time. But it's not just the discomfort you need to worry about. You also need to check your health well.

If you don't know, being obese or overweight can lead to a number of dangerous diseases like diabetes, high blood pressure, kidney disease, cardiovascular disease, stroke, and even cancer. And unfortunately, there are so many people in the world who are clearly overweight these days.

This level of inactivity for the modern human being can be very damaging to health. This is why it is necessary for people to really commit to a rigid and effective exercise routine. To compensate for the level of inactivity that is undertaken during the rest of the day, it is necessary to dedicate a few minutes or hours to even just a rigorous physical activity. So, this requires asking the question, what constitutes exercise?

Remember that regular physical activity is different from exercise. The physical activity you do every day, such as walking to your car or getting up from your desk, is not a form of exercise. Yes, you are exerting a certain amount of effort by recruiting muscles. But it's not necessarily intense physical activity.

Exercise is a more strenuous, planned and focused physical activity. However, exercise can mean different things to many different people, considering we all have varying degrees of fitness level. For an older person who is overweight, walking for 20 minutes could be exercise. However, for a relatively fit 20-year-old, walking for 20 minutes is essentially just regular physical activity. Essentially,

Intensity measurement

You don't have to engage in complex and meticulous quantitative measurements of your physical activity to figure out if you are exercising or not. You just have to pay attention to how you feel. To keep things simple, you can classify intensity into two different categories: moderate and vigorous. If you are doing a movement and are having difficulty breathing but are still able to speak as you do it, then it is moderate in intensity. However, when you really struggle to catch your breath to the point where you can't speak anymore, you are engaged in vigorous intensity. When engaging in active exercise, you should aim for a vigorous level of intensity.

How much exercise do you need to do?

In order for you to truly benefit from exercise, you need to develop a routine for yourself. This routine should get you to do some sort of aerobic or anaerobic exercise at least three times a week. For each of these sessions, you should try to make them last from 30 minutes to an hour. Obviously, the more intense and longer your workout, then the more calories you will be able to actively burn. So, with the additional calories you are burning, the faster you will be able to lose weight.

General tips for exercise
Find a routine you enjoy

You won't train consistently if you hate doing it. So, explore different apps, machines and routines until you find a few that you like. It's okay to stick with those for a while until they get easy or boring. So you can turn it on with something new.

Keep your goal in mind

When you feel too lazy to exercise, it's easy to forget why you're doing it in the first place. Instead of straining to work out, try to visualize what your body will look like and how you will feel after all your efforts.

Start slowly

If you lack motivation to train, don't pester yourself. Set small goals for yourself, just to get used to it. Or tell yourself it's only this once for a few minutes. Once you actually start training, you will feel good thanks to the endorphins it triggers. We advise you to keep the habit.

Set trigger

Your reward center will remember the feeling that comes from a workout. You can trigger the desire for that feeling by leaving your gym clothes or workout gear out. And you're more likely to exercise if you make the process as convenient as possible.

Hydrate

Make sure you are hydrated before training and always have water on you. Dehydration will cause you to burn too quickly.

Stretch

Stretch after your workouts so you don't hurt yourself too much to exercise the next day. Hold each stretch for 20-30 seconds. Start the stretch gently, in a place where it doesn't cause discomfort. Then gradually stretch the muscle even more every few seconds, as it loosens.

To refuel

Refuel after workouts with water and at least one fruit if you're hungry.

Not beyond caffeine

Pre-workouts contain caffeine and amphetamine-like compounds that can damage blood vessels. Some of them have even been withdrawn from the market because they have caused fatal heart disease. Even just having a coffee before a workout can be harmful. Caffeine constricts blood vessels as blood flows through them, which can cause damage.

Strength Training Tips
To breathe

Before starting, take a few deep breaths through your nose and out of your mouth. Once you begin your workout, exhale through your nose as you lift the weight or contract the muscle. Inhale through your nose as you lower the weight or extend the muscle.

Use your head

As you perform this exercise, focus your mind on the muscle you are trying to strengthen. It will keep you focused during your workout and maximize the benefits. Your muscles actually respond to your thoughts. It may sound crazy, but studies have shown that even without any physical movement, strength develops through mental attention to just the muscle.

Increase time under tension

Time under tension refers to how long your muscle is under strain during a set. Straining a muscle for a longer period of time results in increased muscle exhaustion.

In other words, slow down each set to 30-40 seconds each to increase muscle growth.

Maintain a steady pace throughout the set, including the time you are lowering the weight.

rest

Give each muscle group at least one day of rest. And take at least one full day off each week from exercising.

High intensity interval training

If you hate spending time on cardio, try high-intensity interval training. You will burn the same number of calories in less time.

An example of HIIT on the elliptical or treadmill is:

Warm-up on foot for 4 minutes

15 minutes alternating between running for 45 seconds and walking for 45 seconds

4 minutes walk to cool down

Aerobics vs. Anaerobic

While there are many different forms of exercise, they can all ultimately be grouped into one of two categories: aerobic and anaerobic. No particular type of exercise will be better than the other. It so happens that these two categories of exercises have different purposes and impact the body in different ways. To learn more about the differences between aerobic and anaerobic exercise, read on.

Aerobic

Aerobic fitness can also be considered cardiovascular fitness. Basically, aerobic exercise is any type of moderately intense exercise that raises the heart rate and raises the body's core temperature. During aerobic exercise, there is moderate stress on the muscles and heart. Generally, aerobic exercises are more sustainable. It is easier to sustain aerobic exercise for a prolonged duration than anaerobic exercise.

When the body is in an aerobic state, the heart rate increases until it reaches a state of discomfort, but it is not uncomfortable enough to be unable to speak. Aerobic exercises are effective for weight loss because they cause you to burn calories while you are actually performing the movements. Here are some examples of aerobic exercises:

- Running

- I swim

- Skipping rope

- Brisk walking

- Cycling

- Boating

Anaerobic

Anaerobic exercises are generally more intense and cannot be sustained for extended periods of time. Typically, these are comprised of movements that are performed in short bursts at a rapid pace. When your body reaches an anaerobic state, your heart rate becomes so high that you wouldn't really be able to focus on anything other than trying to breathe.

During anaerobic exercise, lactic acid gradually builds up in the muscles and could eventually lead to muscle failure or numbness. Anaerobic exercises are mainly associated with muscle growth and strength gain. This is how they differ from aerobic exercises which focus on endurance, endurance, and overall conditioning. Anaerobic exercises are effective for weight loss because they put the body's metabolism into hyperdrive for up to 48 hours after a training session.

Here are some examples of anaerobic exercises:

- Olympic weightlifting

- Sprint

- High intensity interval training

- CrossFit

- Gym

- Calisthenics

The 10 components of fitness

If you think you can lose weight by being exceptionally good at just two or three components of fitness, then that's fine. However, if you are truly intent on understanding the science of exercise and how you can holistically approach your fitness training, then you need to familiarize yourself with each of these components.

Resistance

Resistance is the human body's ability to absorb, process and deliver oxygen. Whenever you engage in strenuous physical activity, your body will consume more oxygen than is needed than when you are simply resting. So, the more stamina you have, the more your body will be able to keep up with you even as you keep pushing yourself with training and exercise. To train your endurance, you need to engage in a physical activity that elevates your heart rate to a state of discomfort. Hence, you need to keep that elevated heart rate for as long as possible. The key to improving every time is through gradual sensory overload. As your heart strengthens, some physical activities become easier. When that's the case

Resistance

Then comes the resistance. Resistance is actually very similar to resistance in the sense that it has to do with the body's ability to sustain physical movement under pressure and tension. However, while regular resistance is about cardiovascular strength, endurance has more to do with muscle strength. The better your stamina, the more efficient your body will be at breaking down energy sources such as fat and glycogen.

So, to be more concrete, your stamina will be what will allow you to run for two hours without stopping. Your stamina will be what will allow you to sustain sprint intervals at full speed after a short rest period. If you have good stamina, you will be able to recover faster after a burst of energy expenditure.

Power

Power. While this is a word that many people may be familiar with, not too many would be aware of its scientific definition. Your strength is the ability of your muscle units to apply force in a single contraction. As you build your strength, you are able to move more weight and apply more force through the use of muscles. Strength training is done by lifting heavy weights for numerous repetitions. This is an effective training method for fat loss as well because it requires so much from the body's metabolic system. At the same time, strength allows the human body to be able to do more things during workouts.

Power

Strength and power are two components that are often intertwined, and this is because they share some fundamental principles. Strength is determined by the amount of force your muscles are capable of producing. However, your power is determined by how quickly the force generated by your muscles is applied. This is why power is a crucial component in workouts such as Olympic weightlifting, sprinting or boxing. When you are powerful, you are able to exert your strength at a much faster and more efficient rate. This results in better athletic performance.

Agility

Think of a fly in your room that you are desperately trying to chase away but can't seem to. See the fly moving in a certain direction. Beforehand, you try to crush it, but they are able to quickly switch to another unexpected direction to catch you off guard.

This is agility. It is your body's ability to quickly switch from one movement pattern to another. In sports, boxers would be perfect examples of agility. The speed of a boxer to block an opponent's punch and quickly counter it with a punch of his own would be a demonstration of their agility. However, to improve your agility, you need to improve other components of fitness as well. These components are speed, coordination, precision, balance and flexibility. This will be discussed in depth as we head further down this list.

Speed

Speed is your body's ability to reduce the amount of time it takes to perform a repeated movement. If we go back to the boxer example, a manifestation of that boxer's speed would be the number of punches they would be able to repeatedly throw in a given amount of time. Of course, there are other factors that come into play here, such as stamina and endurance. It is not uncommon for some physical components of fitness to intertwine and complement each other. Speed can manifest itself in a number of ways and is one of the most difficult components of fitness to train.

Flexibility

When you think of flexibility, chances are you automatically think of a yogi. Flexibility is the body's ability to maintain strength and control through different planes of motion. As you may already know, your body is made up of several joints and muscles. The more flexible you are, the better you will be at manipulating your body into certain positions without experiencing any pain or extreme discomfort. Flexibility is important in training because it is a good indicator of how prone an athlete might be to injury. The less flexible you are, the more prone you are to injuries surrounding the joints and muscles. In other words, flexibility is your body's ability to bend without breaking.

Equilibrium

Balance is all about control. One of the most important aspects of fitness is the body's ability to control its center of gravity in relation to its support base. Balance is a very important component of fitness for athletes such as skateboarders, skiers, surfers, gymnasts, martial artists and more. Balance is classified more in neurological form than physical form, as it largely has to do with the brain's power to send signals to focal points in the body. However, while not many athletes notice this, balance plays a very important role in the efficiency of simple movements like running and jumping. Coordination

Coordination is the ability to maintain composure and control while simultaneously performing several movement patterns at the same time. For dancers, coordination is key. While the left arm performs a particular pattern of movement, a dancer must also master the art of having the right leg perform a different pattern of movement. Like balance, coordination is also classified under the neurological form. It is something that can only be trained through pure repetition and practice.

Precision

Finally, there is the accuracy. To put it simply, precision is the body's ability to control its movements with precision and direction at varying intensities. Accuracy is a fundamental component of fitness for basketball players. In order for a basketball player's biomechanics to translate into a scored basket, the accuracy in shooting the basketball is equivalent. And as you may have guessed, precision is also a neurological skill, just like balance and coordination.

Benefits of Exercise

Yes, exercise is a very powerful tool that you can use to help you lose weight. However, in addition to serving as a valuable tool for losing weight, regular exercise and physical activity will also offer you other health benefits. Of course, not many people would be too thrilled with the idea of sweating and getting dirty from exercising several times a week. Some individuals will need a little more persuasion than others. If you need to be further enticed to adopt an exercise routine for yourself, read on. Here are the other benefits of exercise besides weight loss:

You have more energy

Whenever you exercise regularly, you will see some huge improvements in your overall fitness. This partly means that your stamina and endurance will improve as well. Your stamina and endurance are responsible for having the energy to do the things you do every day. So, if you train constantly, you are also increasing your work capacity. When you have more energy, you end up becoming more focused, driven, motivated and productive in life. You will simply begin to feel that you have so much more energy to do more things. This energy will serve as fuel to achieve your ambitions and goals.

Sleep better at night

Not many people realize that one of the greatest benefits of exercise is getting a good night's sleep. Think about it. As a human being, your body is always ready to generate a lot of energy to sustain itself. It foresees that you have a lot of things to do during the day and then prepares an energy harvest to use. For many people who are inactive, there is a lot of pent-up energy within them that doesn't run out and stays with them until the night. Here's how exercise can help people sleep better. When you use that energy by engaging in strenuous physical activity, you will deplete the sources of energy your body is producing. This will lead to better sleep quality at night.

Get a boost in endorphins

Endorphins, otherwise known as happiness hormones, will always be in full abundance for people who exercise regularly. Whenever you exercise, your brain triggers the release of chemicals called endorphins in your body. Endorphins are responsible for improving your mood and making you feel lighter and more optimistic about life. So, every time you work out, you're essentially giving yourself a natural endorphin high. You are generating a good mood for yourself. This is why it is also a great idea for people to work out whenever they feel stressed, anxious or angry. The release of endorphins can do wonders for a person's mood.

You've improved your sex life

While for many people sex is a very emotional (and possibly spiritual) act, it still has a large physical component. To have a thriving sex life, you need to achieve a certain level of fitness as well. You need to have strength, stamina, endurance, and even flexibility if you really want to maximize the fun you have in your bedroom. These are all things you get better at every time you train and train regularly. Additionally, sweat is known to be a natural aphrodisiac. You have a lot to gain in the bedroom from working out in the gym.

You just feel better about yourself

Finally, you end up feeling better about yourself after a workout. Of course, when you train constantly, you are also chiseling your physique. The physical changes that take place in your body will give you a renewed sense of confidence and self-worth. Plus, whenever you hit certain fitness milestones, you become proud of that sense of accomplishment. Overall, you end up being more proud of who you are as a person every time you train. You become much more comfortable and comfortable with who you are.

You don't have to set goals for yourself to be a professional athlete. It is not necessary. The point here is that you understand how you can best speed up your weight loss journey. And the answer is that you have a solid and reliable training program that you enjoy doing and can support. This is really the point. Of course, you can be proud of yourself for going out and running for an hour. However, if you don't like running and don't see the point, it would be really hard for you to support it as a training program.

At the end of the day, the only important thing here is that you understand why it is important for you to exercise. You have simply been given the tools you need to motivate you to start being more active. If you're still having trouble determining which type of workout routine would be right for you, don't worry.

CHAPTER 6:

Frequently asked questions about the Optavia diet

You may have some questions about the Optavia diet plan. Below are some of the common frequently asked questions people ask about this diet.

Which program is right for me?

Optavia offers a wide variety of programs designed to improve health and well-being. Choosing the right one is easy as these diet plans are designed for different individuals and their needs. However, if you are still unsure which diet to follow, you can always get in touch with an Optavia trainer to learn about the many options you have.

Is it okay for me to skip supplies?

Refueling is very important as it is specifically formulated with the right balance of macronutrients (carbohydrates, fats and proteins). Proper fueling can help promote an efficient fat burning state so that people lose fat without losing their energy. If you skip your refueling, you could be missing out on these important nutrients, including your daily allowance of vitamins and minerals. Now, if you accidentally skip your supplies within 24 hours, doubling down is crucial so you don't lose the nutrition your supplies provide.

What is the best plan for my fitness level?

Exercise can lead to permanent transformation. This is why a specific Optavia diet program is designed for people who have different levels of activity.

Active adults who engage in 45 minutes of light to moderate exercise can benefit from Plan 5 & 1. Always talk to your coach about which plan is best for your age and activity level.

Can I rearrange my supplies, especially if I work long days or night duty?

Yes. You can rearrange the timing of your replenishment, depending on your schedule. What's important is consuming your lean, green supplies and meals within 24 hours. So whether you work at night or at regular hours, make sure you eat your meals every 2 to 3 hours for as long as you are awake.

How often should I eat my meals?

The Optavia diet plan teaches you the habit of eating healthy. You are encouraged to have six small meals a day. As mentioned above, you are encouraged to eat every two to three hours after waking up. So, start the day with supplies and eat your lean, green meals in between your supplies. It is recommended to consume the first meal within one hour of waking up to ensure optimal blood sugar. This is also a good hunger control strategy.

Can I dine out during the Optavia diet program?

Meals on special days are simpler than you would expect! Simply rearrange your replenishment schedule so you can celebrate your lean, green food at your morning reunion, family picnic, banquet ceremony, family restaurant dinner, or just about any unique meal occasion!

Depending on your lean options, you can have your usual lean, green meal consisting of 5 to 7 ounces of prepared lean protein, three amounts of non-starchy veggies, and 0-2 amounts of good fat.

Request that your meat be prepared / served without sauces and / or processed fats; turn off starchy plant alternatives (like potatoes) for reduced carbohydrate choices (like steamed green beans or broccoli). Ask your waiter to lose the bread basket or cup of chips and instead keep the salad dressing on the floor.

If you can't resist the consumption of foods that are not part of the lean and green diet, you will increase your regular calorie consumption, so starting with the next diet;

you will return to the Optavia program. And if you think you've eaten too much, it's always best not to skip meals. Get ahead with your strategy as fast as possible.

Alternatively, when dining out, you should bring a Fueling with you and ask the restaurant for cold or hot water (depending on what you eat) to match your Fueling. So prepare your food and enjoy it like everyone else!

You have, as you can see, some choices. Be sure to email your Opotavia Mentor for further help and advice.

Which foods do not comply with the Optavia diet?

- Alcohol is not approved during the weight loss process. According to the organization, it provides calories, which leaves you sleepy.

- Remove coconut oil, butter or reduce solids.

- Miss out on cookies and sweets that contain huge calories.

- Keep away from carbonated drinks.

   Do you have direct indications on when, what and how much to consume while on the

Medifast 5 & 1 plan. Especially while going out? Wherever you go, you can continue the menu with balanced lean and green meals, or safe change and maintenance options, almost anywhere. All it takes is a little imagination and preparation. Many restaurants have options that are or may be service compliant with a little tweaking. The most important thing to note is that it is safe to ask questions about "personalizing" the order on your website. Many locations are more than capable of meeting specific needs and can provide alternative replacements for free or for a small price.

Some suggestions: BEFORE you proceed

Study the choices that are plannable, so you know what to look for when selecting!

Search. Review the menu in person or online in-store or call ahead and prepare your order in advance. Deciding WHAT to Buy When determining how to prepare your meals, keep in mind that some ways of cooking add extra calories and fat to the meal. Prepare your meals using one of the suggested techniques to make sure your meal is low in carbohydrates and fat.

Stick to the recommended lean protein and vegetarian options for your Lean & Green meal when you're on the 5 & 1 plan.

Foods prepared this way are right for you.	Foods to avoid that are prepared this way. (It's not right for you.)

Fresh garden	Sauce
Boiled	Buttery or buttery
Grilled	Crispy, fried (all kinds of fried foods)
Roasted	Cream sauce or cream

Keep food "naked", including missing or walking condiments, dressings or sauces.

Use tenderloin (sirloin) or circular cuts when eating beef and always remove some noticeable fat from the product.

Continue for water-based soups. Cream soups (not including Medifast cream soups) appear to be high in calories.

The healthiest type of sauce is olive oil, marinara or tomato sauce.

"Low carbohydrate" does not simply imply "low calorie" or "low fat". Make sure you read the label carefully and decide if a low-carb item is the right food option.

Select whole grain products, such as brown bread, pasta, and brown rice.

Grilled	In cheese sauce
In shirt	In Butter or Oil
Steamed	Breaded or with Scampi
Charbroiled	Scalloped
	Pastry
	Coconut milk or peanut sauce

Chapter 7
Optavia Air Fryer Recipes

1. Mustard Chicken Nuggets With Honey

1 Lean │ 1 Replenishment │ 2 Condiments
Preparation time: 5 minutes │ Cooking time: 20 minutes │ Servings: 2

Ingredients:

Chicken Breast, Skinless, Boneless, Cubed - 12 oz

Egg, beaten - 1

Honey and onion mustard sticks - 2 sachets

Plain, low-fat Greek yogurt - ¼ cup

Brown, spicy mustard - 2 tsp

Ground garlic - ¼ tsp

Cooking spray - just enough

Indications:
1. Wash the chicken and dry it.
2. Mash the honey mustard and onion sticks to a breadcrumb consistency in a shallow bowl.
3. Preheat the air fryer to 205 ° C.
4. Keep the beaten egg and the chopped honey mustard and onion stick in two separate shallow bowls.
5. Line aluminum foil in the pan of the air fryer and lightly grease it with cooking spray.
6. Take the boneless chicken cubes one by one, dip them in honey and sprinkle them with the honey mustard and onion stick powder and pour onto the pan.
7. Repeat whole chicken cubes.
8. Cook the chicken for 20 minutes, turning it intermittently until the core temperature of the meat reaches 75 ° C.
9. While cooking, mix the garlic powder, Greek yogurt, and mustard in a small bowl to make the sauce.
10.   Serve the nugget with the sauce.
Nutritional values per serving:
Calories: 364 | Fat: 6.8 g | Cholesterol: 181 mg | Sodium: 408 mg | Carbohydrates:

24 g | Protein: 49 g

2. Salmon burger with green salad

1 Lean │3 Green │3 Condiments │ ½ Snack
Preparation time: 10 minutes | Cooking
time: 13 minutes | Servings: 2

Ingredients:

For the salmon burgers:
   Canned Pink Salmon, Boneless - 5 oz

   Egg - 1

   Mayonnaise, light - 1 and a half
   tablespoons

   Lemon juice - ½ tsp

   Onion, finely grated - 1 tbsp

   Parsley, dried - ¼ tsp

   Pepper, ground - ¼ tsp

   Multigrain Crackers, Mashed - 10 oz

Cooking spray - just enough

For the salad:

Cucumber, peeled and sliced - 3 cups.

Regular, Low Fat Greek Yogurt - 3 oz

Apple cider vinegar - 2 tbsp

Dill, fresh - 1 tbsp

Pepper - ¼ tsp

Salt - ¼ tsp

Indications:
1. Drain the salmon well 2. Beat the egg in a small bowl.
Combine mayonnaise, egg, onion, lemon juice, pepper, and parsley in a medium bowl to make a smooth paste.
Put the crushed and chopped salmon inside and gently fold the mixture.
Make the mixture into two meatballs.
Sprinkle some cooking on the pan of the air fryer and place the meatballs on top.
Set the temperature to 190 ° C and cook for 13 minutes turning the sides intermittently.

8. While cooking, in a medium bowl, gently mix the vinegar, yogurt, dill, pepper and salt.
9. Add the sliced cucumber and mix gently.
10. Serve the salmon burger with the salad.

Nutritional values per serving:
Calories: 294 | Fat: 12.9 g | Cholesterol: 118 mg | Sodium: 470 mg | Carbohydrates: 19 g | Protein: 24 g

3. Egg and vanilla smoothie

⅓ Lean | 1 Replenishment | 1½ Condiments
Preparation time: 5 minutes | Cooking time: 5 minutes | Servings: 2

Ingredients:

Optavia Essential Creamy Vanilla Shake - 2 sachets (1.13 oz / sachet)

Vanilla Almond Milk, Unsweetened - 16 oz

Pasteurized eggs; separated yolk - 2

Rum extract - ½ tsp

Nutmeg - ¼ tsp

Indications:

1. In an air fryer compatible cooking bowl, combine the rum extract, vanilla smoothie, and vanilla almond milk.
2. Place the intestines in the air fryer and heat for 5 minutes at 205 ° C.
3. Take it out and transfer it to a blender.
4. Add the egg yolk and blend until smooth.
5. Put the egg white in a small bowl and beat it with a hand blender until it begins to foam.
6. Transfer the beaten egg to a large glass.
7. Pour over the vanilla smoothie mixture and sprinkle with a pinch of nutmeg. 8. Serve cool

Nutritional value per serving:

Calories: 404 │ Fat: 11.5 g │ Cholesterol: 212 mg │ Sodium: 227 mg │ Carbohydrates:

45 g │ Protein: 11 g

4.   Peanut   Butter Chocolate Donuts

1 Refueling | 1 Seasoning | ½ Snack Optional

Preparation time: 10 minutes | Cooking time: 15 minutes | Servings: 2

Ingredients:

Optavia Essential Golden Chocolate Chip Pancakes - 3 oz

Optavia Essential Decadent Double Chocolate Brownie - 3 oz

Liquid egg substitute - 3 tbsp

Unsweetened Vanilla Almond Milk - ⅛ cup

Vanilla extract - ¼ tsp

Baking powder - ¼ tsp

Cooking spray - just enough

For the glaze:

Peanut butter, ground - ¼ cup

Vanilla almond milk, unsweetened - 2 tbsp

Indications:

1. Preheat the air fryer to 175 ° C.
2. Place the chocolate pancake shavings in a bowl and crumble.
3. Combine brownies, milk, egg substitute, vanilla extract, and yeast.
4. Sprinkle some cooking oil on the crevices of the donuts.
5. Transfer the mixture evenly into the 4 slots of the donut pan.
6. Place the pan in the air fryer and bake for 15 minutes until it turns well.
7. After that, take it out of the deep fryer and let it cool for the glaze.
8. For the frosting, combine the ground peanut butter and milk in a shallow bowl until smooth and thin.
9. Dip the donuts in the glaze and decorate with chocolate chips.
10. Serve cool.

Nutritional values per serving:
Calories: 397 │ Fat: 14.7 g │ Cholesterol: 4 mg │ Sodium: 430 mg │ Carbohydrates:

63 g │ Protein: 7 g

5. sweet potato muffins

1 Refueling | ½ Condiments | Half a portion of lean
Preparation time: 5 minutes | Cooking time: 15 minutes Servings: 2

Ingredients:

Optavia Honey Sweet Potatoes - 1 sachet (31g)

Egg whisk - 2 tbsp

Baking powder - ¼ tsp

Water - ½ cup

Ground cinnamon - ⅛ tsp

Cooking spray - just enough

Muffin cups - 2

Indications:

1. Preheat the air fryer to 180 ° C.
2. In a medium bowl, combine the egg whisk, sweet potato, yeast, and water well.

3. Sprinkle some cooking oil into the muffin cups.
4. Pour the mixture evenly into the muffin cups.
5. Sprinkle ground cinnamon on top.
6. Place the muffin tins in the air fryer and bake for 15 minutes at 180 ° C.
7. After 15 minutes, remove and serve hot.

Nutritional values per serving:
Calories: 24 | Fat: 0.1 g | Cholesterol: 0 mg | Sodium: 38 mg | Carbohydrates: 4 g | Protein: 2 g

6.   sticks of French toast

1 Refueling | 3 Condiments
Preparation time: 5 minutes | Cooking time: 4 minutes | Servings: 2

Ingredients:

Optavia Essential Cinnamon Crunchy O's Cereal - 2 sachets (30g x 2)

Cream cheese, low-fat, softened - 2 tbsp

Liquid egg substitute - 6 tbsp

Sugar-free syrup - 2 tbsp

Cooking spray - just enough

Indications:
1. In a blender, blend Cinnamon Crunchy O's until its consistency takes on the appearance of breadcrumbs.
2. Pour the liquid egg substitute and cream cheese into the blender mixture until it turns into a paste.
3. Make 6 French toasts like sticks from the dough.
4. Lightly brush the air fryer grill with oil.
5. Place the French Toast Dough on the wire rack.
6. Set the temperature to 204 ° C and air fry for 4 minutes.
7. After air frying, serve garnished with sugar-free syrup.

Nutritional values per serving:
Calories: 92 | Total Fat: 2.9 g | Cholesterol: 14 mg | Sodium: 215 mg

| Coal: 8 g | Protein: 7 g

7. Buffalo cauliflower wings

1 Replenishment | 3 Greens | 3 Seasonings | 1 Healthy Fat

Preparation time: 10 minutes | Cooking time: 27 minutes | Servings: 2

Ingredients:

Optavia Buttermilk Cheddar Herb Biscuit - 2 sachets

Water - ½ cup

Cauliflower florets - 3 cups

Hot buffalo sauce - ¼ cup

Butter, softened - ½ tbsp

Plain, low-fat Greek yogurt - ¼ cup

Ranch dressing, dry - 1 tsp

Cooking spray - just enough

Indications:

Set the air fryer to 220 ° C and preheat.

2. Combine the buttermilk cheddar herb cookie and water in a medium bowl.
3. To this, add the cauliflower flowers and mix well to get good coverage.
4. Line a foiled baking sheet on the cooking tray of the air fryer.
5. Lightly sprinkle cooking oil on the parchment paper.
6. Place the coated cauliflower florets on the aluminum foil.
7. Set the timer for 20 minutes and bake.
8. Now make the sauce and butter by mixing the hot sauce and butter in a medium bowl.
9. Dip the florets in the oven and place them back on the aluminum foil in the air fryer.
10. Now bake for another 7 minutes, shaking intermittently to fry evenly.
11. To make the ranch sauce, combine the ranch mixture and yogurt in a small bowl.
12. Serve the buffalo cauliflower wings with ranch sauce.

Nutritional values per serving:
Calories: 266 | Fat: 7.8 g | Cholesterol: 6 mg | Sodium: 801 mg | Carbohydrates: 41 g

| Protein: 10 g

8. Lobster roll in romaine lettuce

1 Leaner │3 Green │1 Seasoning │2 Healthy fats

Preparation time: 10 minutes │ Cooking time: 4 minutes │ Servings: 2

Ingredients:

Lobster meat, cooked - 6 ounces romaine lettuce, small - 1 butter, melted - ½ tbsp.

Greek yogurt, plain, low fat - ½ cup

Mayonnaise with olive oil base - 1 tbsp

Celery, small stalk, diced - 1

Lemon juice - 1 tsp

Chives, fresh, chopped - ½ tbsp

Old Bay seasoning - ¼ tsp

Pepper, ground - ¼ tsp

Salt - ⅛ tsp

Indications:

1. Preheat the air fryer to 190 ° C.
2. Cut the romaine hearts in half lengthwise.
3. Make a little boat-shaped lobster filling by removing some of the inside leaves of the romaine hearts.
4. Apply some butter to the inside of the boat-shaped portion of the Roman leaves.
5. Place the coated lettuce in the pan of the air fryer and select the grill at 190 ° C for 3-4 minutes to get slightly charred and taste like lettuce.
6. Mix all ingredients, except the lobster meat, in a large bowl.
7. Now gently fold all of the lobster in until the mixture is covered with lobster.
8. Evenly distribute the covered lobster in the boat-shaped lettuce.
9. Serve and enjoy.

Nutritional values per serving:
Calories: 176 │ Fat: 6.1 g │ Cholesterol: 117 mg │ Sodium: 591 mg │ Carbohydrates:

8 g │ Protein: 23 g

9. Salmon with cucumber, dill and tomato salad

1 Lean │ 3 Green │ 3 Condiments
Preparation time: 10 minutes │ Cooking time: 10 minutes │ Servings: 2

Ingredients:

Salmon - ¾ lb.

Cucumber, sliced - 2 cups

Cherry Tomatoes, Halved - 8 oz.

Cider vinegar - ⅛ cup

Dill, fresh, chopped - ⅛ cup

Salt - ⅛ tsp

Pepper, ground - ⅛ tsp

Za'atar - ½ tbsp

Lemon wedges - 2 lemons

Indications:

1. Set the air temperature to 180 ° C and preheat.

2. Put the cucumber, tomatoes, vinegar, dill, salt and pepper in a medium bowl and mix to mix well.
3. Rub Za'atar over the salmon and let it cook for 3-4 minutes.
4. Line the pan of the air fryer with parchment paper.
5. Place the seasoned salmon on top without overlapping it.
6. Cook for 10 minutes, turning the sides in half.
7. Serve hot with salad.
8. Top it with lemon wedges.

Nutritional values per serving:
Calories: 304 | Fat: 8.2 g | Cholesterol: 78 mg | Sodium: 212 mg | Carbohydrates: 21 g | Protein: 37 g

10. Turkey meat with fennel

1 Lean | 3 Green | 3 Condiments | 2 Healthy fats
Preparation time: 10 minutes | Cooking time: 36 minutes | Servings: 2

Ingredients:

Lean turkey, ground - ¾ lb.

Cabbage, finely chopped - 1 and a half cups

Onion, green, finely chopped - 1

Toasted pine nuts, chopped - ⅛ cup

Paprika - 1 tsp

Salt, divided - 1 tsp

Pepper, coarsely, crushed, divided - 1 tsp

Olive oil - ½ tsp

Fennel bulb, small - ½ lb.

Grated Parmesan - 1 tbsp

Indications:

Wash the turkey and drain it with a colander.
Preheat the air fryer to 205 ° C for 10 minutes.
Combine the chopped turkey meat, chopped cabbage, pine nuts, half the salt, chopped onion and half pepper in a large bowl.

4. In the air fryer tray, roll out parchment paper and place the turkey meat mix and turn it into a 7 "x 4" sized loaf of bread.
5. Place the pan in the oven with air fryer.
6. At 205 ° C, bake the meatloaf for 30 minutes until the internal temperature of the meat reaches 75 ° C.
7. Once cooked, remove it and keep it ready to use.
8. Now start working the fennel.
9. Remove the fennel stalks and cut them in half lengthwise.
10. Cut the halves again and remove the core.
11. Lightly apply olive oil to the basket of the air fryer.
12. Place the chopped fennel bulbs on top and fry for 6 minutes at 180 ° C until they become tender and lightly golden.
13. Once they become tender, transfer them to a serving dish.
14. Season the remaining salt, pepper and mix gently.
15. Now slice the fried turkey loaf and place it on top of the fried fennel.
16. Sprinkle with grated Parmesan and serve hot.

Nutritional values per serving:

Calories: 305 | Fat: 8 g | Cholesterol: 99 mg | Sodium: 1440 mg | Carbohydrates: 15 g | Protein: 44 g

11.Grilled chicken with green dressing

1 Lean |3 Green |3 Condiments |1 Healthy Fat

Preparation time: 15 minutes | Cooking time: 20 minutes | Servings: 2

Ingredients:

Chicken breast, skinless and boneless - ¾ lbs.

Salt - ¼ tsp

Pepper - ¼ tsp

Kabocha squash, diced - ½ cup

Zucchini, finely chopped - ½ cup

Summer squash, finely chopped - ½

cup
broccoli,
finely
chopped - ½
cup   cherry
tomatoes,
cut in half -
4 nos.

Radishes, thinly sliced - 4 n.

Red cabbage, finely chopped - ½ cup.

For the green dressing:
Low-fat Greek yogurt - ¼ cup chopped fresh
basil - ½ cup.
Clove of garlic - 1

Lemon juice - 2 tbsp

Ground pepper - ¼ tsp

Salt - ¼ tsp

Indications:
1. Preheat the air fryer to 180 ° C.
2. Season the chicken with pepper and salt in a
   shallow bowl.

3. Place the chicken in the air fryer and roast for 12-15 minutes.
4. When the internal temperature of the chicken reaches 75 ° C, remove it on a cutting board and cut it into small pieces.
5. Now in a baking dish, place the chopped yellow summer squash, kabocha squash, broccoli and zucchini.
6. Cook them in the air fryer for 5 minutes until tender.
7. Now make the green dressing by blending the green dressing in a blender until they become a smooth puree.
8. To serve, place the vegetables on a serving dish and arrange the sliced cherry tomatoes, radishes, chopped cabbage and chicken.
9. Top it with green dressing.

Nutritional values per serving:
Calories: 334 | Total fat: 16 g | Cholesterol: 109 mg | Sodium: 415 mg | Carbohydrates: 10 g | Protein: 37 g

12.   Spinach   and zucchini   in   the Optavia air fryer

1 Lean │ 3 Green │ 1 Seasoning
Preparation time: 10 minutes │ Cooking time: 25 minutes │ Servings: 2

Ingredients: Spinach - ½ cup

Zucchini - 1 large

Skimmed cottage cheese - ½ cup.

Egg - 1

Mozzarella, grated, divided - ¾ cup

Grated Parmesan - ¼ cup

Tomato sauce, a little sugar - ¼ cup

Salt - ⅛ tsp

Nutmeg - ⅛ tsp

Cooking oil - just enough

Parchment

Direction:
1. Preheat the air fryer to 190 ° C.
2. Julien zucchini cut into thin slices and keep them ready for use.

3. Combine the egg, ricotta, half of the grated mozzarella, spinach, Parmesan, nutmeg, and salt in a medium bowl.
4. Place parchment paper in the pan and sprinkle cooking oil on it.
5. Arrange the courgette slices in two sets, stacking them on a plate.
6. Place the ricotta mixture at the end of the courgette slice and roll up.
7. Now place the rolled courgettes on parchment paper.
8. Over the zucchini pour the tomato sauce.
9. Sprinkle with grated cheese and bake for 25 minutes.
10. Serve hot.

Nutritional value per serving:
Calories: 350 | Fat: 17 g | Cholesterol: 359 mg | Sodium: 1197 mg | Carbohydrates: 18 g | Protein: 31 g

13. Pork chops in spinach salad

1 Lean | 3 Green | 3 Condiments
Preparation time: 10 minutes | Cooking time: 12 minutes | Servings: 2

Ingredients:

Pork Chops - 2 (14 oz)

Lime juice - 1 tsp

Seasoning in jerky - ½ tbsp

Salt - ½ tsp

Baby Spinach - 4 cups Radishes - ½ cup
Diced tomato - ½ cup
Lemon juice - ½ tbsp
Ground black pepper - ½ tsp

Indications:
1. Wash the pork and drain it.
2. Season with salt, jerk dressing, lime juice and marinate for about 30 minutes in a medium bowl.
3. Place the marinated pork chops in the air fryer.
4. Set the temperature to 230 ° C and bake for 12 minutes until the core temperature of the meat reaches 65 ° C.
5. Meanwhile, boil the water in a small bowl and put the spinach in it.
6. Remove it on a plate when it wilts.
7. Put the radishes, tomatoes on the spinach and sprinkle with salt.
8. Transfer the cooked ribs to the vegetables.
9. Serve hot.

Nutritional values per serving:
Calories: 349 | Total fat: 8.6 g |
Cholesterol: 159 mg | Sodium: 1508 mg |
Carbohydrates: 6 g | Protein: 61 g

14. Chicken and salad

1 Lean | 3 Green | 3 Condiments | 1 Healthy Fat

Preparation time: 15 minutes | Cooking time: 25 minutes | Servings: 2

Ingredients:

For the chicken:

Chicken breast, boneless and skinless - ¾ lbs.

Butter, melted - ¾ tbsp

Ground pepper - ¼ tsp

Salt - ¼ tsp

For the salad:

Lettuce, coarsely chopped - 3 cups.

Cucumber, green, sliced - ½ cup

Cherry Tomatoes, Halved - 8 oz

Kalamata pitted olives - 5

Feta cheese, low fat - ¼ cup

Lemon juice - 1 tbsp

Pepper - ¼ tsp

Salt - ¼ tsp

Indications:
1. Wash the chicken and dry it.
2. Preheat the air fryer to 180 ° C.
3. Season the chicken with salt, pepper, butter and let it marinate for 15 minutes.
4. Place the marinated chicken in the grill of the fryer and roast for 25 minutes until the internal temperature of the chicken reaches 70 ° C.
5. After cooking, remove it on a cutting board and let it settle on the fire.
6. Now combine all the salad ingredients in a large bowl and mix well.
7. Slice the chicken and place it on top of the salad.
8. Serve hot.

Nutritional values per serving:
Calories: 406 | Fat: 14.4 g | Cholesterol:
167 mg | Sodium: 734 mg | Carbohydrates:

10 g | Protein: 58 g

15. Gingerbread with cream cheese frosting

1 Refueling | 2 Condiments | 1 Healthy fat
Preparation time: 5 minutes | Cooking 20
minutes | Servings: 2

Ingredients:

Optavia Essential Spiced Gingerbread - 2
sachets

Water - 4 tbsp

Whipped cream cheese with reduced fat
content - 4 tbsp

Vanilla extract - ½ tsp

Liquid stevia - 8 drops

Cooking spray - just enough

Indications:

1. Preheat the air fryer to 175 ° C.
2. Mix the Optavia essential spiced gingerbread and water in a bowl until it becomes a smooth paste.
3. Place a baking sheet on the air fryer basket and sprinkle some cooking oil.
4. Using a baking spoon, make 6 gingersnaps on the greased baking sheet.
5. Set the timer for 20 minutes and air fry until crisp.
6. After cooking, let it cool.
7. To make the glaze, combine the vanilla extract, cream cheese and stevia.
8. Serve the gingerbread with vanilla cheese frosting.

Nutritional values per serving:
Calories: 182 | Total Fat: 5.9 g | Cholesterol: 8 mg | Sodium: 418 mg

| Carbohydrates: 28 g | Protein: 4 g

16. Pepperoni Pizza with Cauliflower Crust

1 Lean │3 Green │3 Condiments
Preparation time: 5 minutes │ Cooking time: 35 minutes │ Servings: 2

Ingredients:

Cauliflower, rice - 2 cups

Mozzarella, low-fat, grated, divided - 1 1/2 cups

Grated Parmesan - ¼ cup

Egg - 1

Italian dressing - ½ tsp

Salt - ¼ tsp

Tomato sauce, sugar-free - ½ cup

Turkey peppers - 10 sticks

Cooking spray - just enough

Indications:

1. Preheat the air fryer to 220 ° C for 10 minutes.
2. Place the cauliflower rice in the pan of the air fryer and saute for 5 minutes, shaking frequently until tender.
3. After that, remove to a shallow bowl and add half of the grated mozzarella, egg, grated Parmesan, salt and Italian seasoning. Gently combine it to mix.
4. Place parchment paper in the pan of the air fryer.
5. Sprinkle some cooking oil and spread the mixture into a round shape in half an inch thick.
6. Cook it in the air fryer for 20 minutes until the edges begin to brown.
7. Once done, garnish the crust with the tomato sauce.
8. Sprinkle the remaining mozzarella on.
9. On top, sprinkle the slices of peppers.
10. Continue cooking for 10 minutes until the cheese begins to melt.
11. Once done, remove it from the air fryer, cut into equal pieces, and serve hot.

Nutritional values per serving:

Calories: 462 | Fat: 8.8 g | Cholesterol: 203 mg | Sodium: 2205 mg | Carbohydrates: 24 g | Protein: 69 g

17. Florentine-style salmon

1 Lean | 3 Green | 3 Condiments
Preparation time: 5 minutes | Cooking time: 19 minutes | Servings: 2

Ingredients:

Salmon fillets - 2½ oz.

Onion, chopped - ¼ cup

Olive oil - 1 tsp

Clove of garlic, finely grated - 1

Spinach, fresh, chopped - 6 oz

Cherry tomatoes, diced - ¾ cup

Red pepper, crushed - ¼ tsp

Pepper, ground - ¼ tsp

Salt - ¼ tsp

Cooking spray - just enough

Indications:

1. Preheat the air fryer to 180 ° C for 10 minutes.
2. Wash the fish fillet and dry it.
3. In a pan suitable for the fryer, fry the chopped onion sprinkled with cooking oil, shaking the container intermittently, until tender at 180 ° C for about 5 minutes.
4. Now add the minced garlic, minced red pepper, minced spinach, ground pepper, salt and diced cherry tomatoes.
5. Fry for about 3-4 minutes, stirring occasionally until the vegetables are soft.
6. Remove it from the pot and let it settle over the heat.
7. Line the pan of the air fryer with parchment paper and spray with cooking oil.
8. Place the fillet on top and place the spinach ricotta on top.
9. Cook the fillet for 15 minutes, until the salmon is well cooked.
10.   Serve hot.
Nutritional values per serving:

Calories: 107 | Fat: 3.9 g | Cholesterol: 26 mg | Sodium: 185 mg | Carbohydrates: 10 g | Protein: 9 g

18. Maple mustard glazed salmon

1 Lean | 3 Condiments | 2 Healthy fats
Preparation time: 5 minutes | Cooking time: 20 minutes | Servings: 2

Ingredients:

Salmon fillet, cut into 4 equal parts - ¾ lb.

Fish broth - ¼ cup

Pancake syrup - ¼ cup

Grainy mustard - 1 tbsp

Soy sauce, low in sodium - ½ tablespoon of ground pepper - ½ tsp

Spray cooking oil - just enough.

Indications:
1. Wash and dry the salmon fillet.
2. In the plate of the air fryer, spray cooking oil and arrange the fillets.
3. Combine the maple syrup, soy sauce, butter, and mustard in a small bowl.
4. Pour the mixture over the salmon fillets.
5. Season some ground pepper on top.
6. Select the cooking option in the air fryer and set the temperature to 220 ° C.
7. Set the timer for 20 minutes and start cooking.
8. It must be ready and check with a fork if it falls apart.
9. Serve hot.

Nutritional values per serving:
Calories: 333 | Fat: 8.7 g | Cholesterol: 78 mg | Sodium: 404 mg | Carbohydrates: 27 g | Protein: 36 g

19. Baked chicken, Italian style

1 Lean │2 Green │3 Condiments │1 Healthy Fat

Preparation time: 5 minutes │ Cooking time: 30 minutes │ Servings: 2

Ingredients:

Shredded Chicken - 10 oz

Ground garlic - ½ tsp

Italian dressing - ½ tsp

Tomato sauce, low carb - 1 cup

Cream cheese - 4 tbsp

Greek yogurt, plain, low fat - ½ cup

Grated Parmesan - ¼ cup

Cooking spray - just enough

Indications:

1. Wash the chopped chicken and drain it through a sieve.
2. Preheat the air fryer to 180 ° C for 10 minutes.

3. Spray cooking oil on the bottom of the air fryer tray.
4. Place the shredded chicken in the air fryer tray.
5. In a small bowl, mix all the ingredients except the tomato sauce.
6. Pour the mixture over the chicken.
7. On top, sprinkle the grated Parmesan.
8. Cook for 30 minutes until the bubble begins.
9. Remove from the air fryer and serve hot.

Nutritional values per serving:
Calories: 399 | Fat: 23.9 g | Cholesterol: 160 mg | Sodium: 520 mg | Carbohydrates: 12 g | Protein: 36 g

20.Baked Broccoli Cheddar Breakfast

1 Lean | 3 Green | 1½ Condiments
Preparation time: 5 minutes | Cooking time: 51 minutes | Servings: 2

Ingredients:
Broccoli florets, small - 3 cups

Water - 3 tbsp

Eggs - 4

Almond milk, unsweetened - ½ cup

Pepper, ground - ¼ tsp

Salt - ¼ tsp

Cayenne pepper, ground - ¼ tsp

Cheddar Cheese, Low Fat, Grated - 2 oz

Cooking spray - just enough

Indications:
In the pan of the air fryer, pour 3 tablespoons of water and insert the broccoli.
Set the temperature to 200 ° C and air fry for 6 minutes.
Transfer the cooked broccoli to a bowl and discard any excess water.
In a mixing bowl, combine the almond milk, eggs, and other seasonings.
Sprinkle some cooking on the pan.
Now place the cooked broccoli in the pan.
Sprinkle the grated cheese over the broccoli and pour the egg and almond mixture over the broccoli.

8. Reset the temperature to 175 ° C and select the cooking option.
9. Set the timer for 45 minutes and bake until the center is solid.
10. Remove it from the air fryer when the top turns light brown.
11. Serve hot.

Nutritional values per serving:
Calories: 164 | Fat: 9.3 g | Cholesterol: 327 mg | Sodium: 338 mg | Carbohydrates: 7 g | Protein: 13 g

21.Bacon Cheeseburger Bites

1 Lean | 1 Green | 3 Condiments
Preparation time: 15 minutes | Cooking time: 18 minutes | Servings: 2

Ingredients:

Lean Ground Beef - ½ lbs.

Yellow onion, finely chopped - ¼ cup

Yellow mustard - 1 tbsp

Clove of garlic, finely grated - 1

Worcestershire sauce - 1 tsp

Salt - ½ tsp

Slice of cheddar cheese, cut into a rectangular shape - 2

Turkey bacon, cooked according to instructions - 2

Dill pickled chips - 12

Lettuce leaves - 4

Halved cherry tomatoes - 6

Cooking spray - just enough

Indications:
Wash the minced meat and drain it well in a colander.
Preheat the air fryer to 205 ° C for 10 minutes.
In a large bowl, combine the thoroughly ground beef, garlic, chopped onion, salt, and Worcestershire sauce.
Make 12 meatballs with the mixture.

5. Line aluminum foil on the air fryer tray.
6. Sprinkle some cooking oil and place the meatballs.
7. Air fry for 15 minutes.
8. Place a piece of cheese on top of each meatball and sauté for another 3 minutes, until the meat begins to melt.
9. When the cheese begins to melt, remove it from the air fryer.
10. Serve the morsels by inserting a toothpick on the meatball and insert the piece of bacon, pickled chips through the toothpick.
11. On top, insert half of the lettuce and tomato to complete the bite of the meatball.
12. Serve and enjoy your bite of meatball.

Nutritional values per serving:
Calories: 123 | Fat: 6.3 g | Cholesterol: 27 mg | Sodium: 353 mg | Carbohydrates: 6 g | Protein: 11 g

22. Baked Spaghetti Squash

1 Lean | 3 Green | 3 Condiments
Preparation time: 5 minutes | Cooking time: 1 hour and 5 minutes | Servings: 2

Ingredients:

Pumpkin spaghetti - 1 medium size

Eggs - 3

Cottage cheese - 1 and a half cups

Sugar substitute, zero calories - 5 sachets

Ground cinnamon - ¼ tsp

Salt - ¼ tsp

Ground nutmeg - ⅛ tsp

Cooking spray - just enough

Indications:
1. Cut the squash in half and remove the seeds.
2. Line the air fryer with aluminum foil and bake the pumpkin face down at 190 ° C for 30 minutes.
3. After 30 minutes, take it out of the air fryer and let it settle on the heat.
4. Pour the spaghetti into a bowl (3 cups).
5. Add all remaining ingredients to the bowl and combine well.
6. Sprinkle some cooking oil into the saucepan and spread the spaghetti mixture.

7. Put it in the air fryer and bake for 35 minutes at 190 ° C until its edge turns golden.
8. After that, remove from the air fryer and let it settle over the heat.
9. Serve hot.

Nutritional values per serving:
Calories: 286 | Fat: 13.3 g | Cholesterol: 272 mg | Sodium: 824 mg | Carbohydrates: 15 g | Protein: 27 g

23. Peanut Butter Cookies

1 Replenishment of | ½ healthy fat | ½ dressings

Preparation time: 15 minutes | Cooking time: 12 minutes | Servings: 2
Ingredients:

Optavia Essential Silky Peanut Butter Shake - 2 sachets

Baking powder - ¼ tsp

Vanilla Almond Milk, unsweetened - ¼ cup

Butter, melted - 1 tsp

Vanilla extract - ¼ tsp

Salt - ⅛ tsp

Cooking spray - just enough

Indications:
1. Preheat the air fryer to 175 ° C.
2. Combine the yeast and peanut butter smoothie in a large bowl.
3. Add the melted butter, vanilla almond milk, vanilla extract and combine well to form a paste. Pour in another tablespoon of milk if necessary.
. Now collect the cookie mixture using a cookie spoon and make 4 cookies.
. Line the pan and drizzle with cooking oil.
. Put the cookies on top.
. With a fork, make a cross mark by pressing lightly on the top of the cookies.
. Season a little salt on the cookies.
. Using the cooking option and bake at 175 ° C for 12 minutes.
0. Serve with unsweetened vanilla milk.

Nutritional values per serving:

Calories: 207 | Fat: 13 g | Cholesterol: 8 mg | Sodium: 268 mg | Carbohydrates: 16 g | Protein: 9 g

24. Cheese Burger Pie

1 Lean | 3 Green | 3 Condiments
Preparation time: 15 minutes | Cooking time: 1 hour 20 minutes | Servings: 2

Ingredients:
Pumpkin Spaghetti - 1 medium lean beef, ground - ½ pound.

Onion, diced - ¼ cup

Eggs - 1

Low-fat Greek yogurt - ½ cup

Tomato puree - 1 tbsp

Worcestershire sauce - ¼ tsp

Cheddar cheese, grated, low fat - ½ cup

Slices of Dill Pickle - 1 oz

Cooking spray - just enough

Indications:

Wash the meat and drain the water completely.

Preheat the air fryer to 200 ° C for 10 minutes.

Cut the spaghetti in half and remove the seeds.

Splash cooking oil inside the pumpkin.

Line the pan with aluminum foil and place the cut side of the pumpkin in front of the foil.

Cook it for 30 minutes.

Take it out of the deep fryer and let it settle over the heat.

Using a fork, scrape the squash to form threads.

Take an air fryer, save the pan and spray it with cooking oil.

Transfer the strands to a cake pan and press them into the pan.

Now, let's make the filling of the cake.

In the plate of the air fryer, fry the meat and onion at 200 ° C for 10 minutes until the meat turns golden.

Stop cooking the air fryer and take it out.

Beat the egg in a medium bowl and combine the tomato paste, Greek yogurt and Worcestershire sauce.

15. Add the cooked meat to the mixture and mix well.
16. Now pour the pie filling over the pumpkin crust.
17. Sprinkle grated cheddar cheese over the pie filling.
18. Decorate with slices of dill pickle.
19. At 200 ° C, bake for 40 minutes.

Nutritional values per serving:
Calories: 515 | Fat: 15.3 g | Cholesterol: 144 mg | Sodium: 786 mg | Carbohydrates: 75 g | Protein: 30 g

25. Roasted vegetables with peanut sauce

1 Lean | 3 Green | 3 Condiments
Preparation time: 10 minutes | Cooking time: 12 minutes | Servings: 2

Ingredients:
Broccoli florets - ¾ cup

Red cabbage, coarsely chopped - ¾ cup.

Pepper, large, cored, halved lengthwise - 1 large

Pepper, ground - ¼ tsp

Salt - ¼

Tofu, ½ "- 1 pound cubes.

Peanut butter, powder - 1 tbsp

Water - 1 ½ tbsp

Sambal - ¼ tbsp

Cooking spray - just enough

Indications:
Wash all the vegetables and dry them.
Preheat the air fryer to 190 ° C.
Place all the vegetables in the pan of the air fryer and lightly drizzle with cooking oil.
Sprinkle with pepper and salt.
Cook the vegetables for 12 minutes, turning them intermittently, until they are caramelized and tender.
Once cooked, remove it in a bowl.
In the pan of the air fryer, stack the tofu cubes and fry at 190 ° C for 15 minutes, turning them intermittently.

8. To make the peanut sauce, combine the peanut powder, sambal, and water in a small bowl.

9. In a serving bowl, place the tofu seasoned with air-fried vegetables.

10. Pour the sauce over the vegetables and serve.

Nutritional values per serving:
Calories: 411 | Fat: 23.1 g | Cholesterol: 0 mg | Sodium: 292 mg | Carbohydrates: 21 g | Protein: 40 g

26. Grilled beef burgers in lettuce wraps

1 Lean | 3 Green | 3 Condiments
Preparation time: 25 minutes | Cooking time: 8 minutes | Servings: 2

Ingredients:

Lean beef, minced - ½ lb.

Salt, divided - 1 tsp

Black pepper, ground, divided - ½ tsp

Garlic, crushed, divided - 1 tsp

Shallot, finely chopped - ½

Capers,
finely
chopped -
½
tablespoon
Feta
cheese, low
fat,
chopped -
1½ oz.

Cucumber, green - ½ pound.

Plain, low-fat Greek yogurt - ¼ cup

Lettuce leaves, large - 4

Cooking spray - just enough

Indications:
Wash and drain the minced meat well with a colander.
In a large bowl, combine the beef with half of the crushed garlic, pepper, and salt.

3. Incorporate the shredded feta into the beef mixture to make 4 equal-sized meatballs and keep it ready.
4. Grate the cucumber, add the remaining salt and combine it.
5. Put the grated cucumber in a colander and let it drain for 10 minutes.
6. Now transfer it to a clean cotton towel and wring out the water as hard as possible.
7. Transfer the squeezed grated cucumber to a medium bowl.
8. Add the remaining salt, garlic, pepper and also add the yogurt.
9. Combine it very well.
10. In the air frying tray, spray cooking oil.
11. Place the meatballs on the pan of the fryer and grill at 190 ° C for 8 minutes by turning the sides intermittently until the core temperature of the meat reaches 75 ° C.
12. Serve the burger on lettuce leaves garnished with cucumber tzatziki.

Nutritional values per serving:
Calories: 246 | Fat: 11.4 g | Cholesterol: 104 mg | Sodium: 1521 mg | Carbohydrates: 6 g | Protein: 31 g

27. Grilled steak in air fryer

1 Lean | 1 Green | 3 Condiments
Preparation time: 10 minutes | Cooking time: 11 minutes | Servings: 2

Ingredients:

Lean Rib Steak - 16 oz

Broccoli - 6 cups

To make the marinade: Beef broth - ¼ cup
Lime juice - 2 tbsp
Cumin, ground - 2 tsp
Coriander, ground - 2 tsp
Clove of garlic, minced - 1
Cooking oil - 2 tbsp

Indications:
Wash the steak and drain the water well.
Mix all the ingredients of the marinade in a blender while slowly adding oil.
Place the steak on a plate and pour the marinade over it.
Refrigerate for 6-8 hours for marinating.
Place the marinated steaks in the pan of the air fryer.

Set the temperature to 205 ° C and grill for 7 minutes, flipping the sides in half and applying the remaining marinade mixture.

After cooking, transfer it to a serving dish.

Now fry the broccoli for 4 minutes, shaking intermittently to also air fry.

Serve the steaks with the broccoli.

Nutritional values per serving:
Calories: 531 │ Fat: 33.8 g │ Cholesterol: 143 mg │ Sodium: 198 mg │ Carbohydrates: 8 g │ Protein: 52 g

28.   Green bean casserole

½ Lean │3 Green │3 Condiments │½ Healthy Fat

Preparation time: 10 minutes │ Cooking time: 47 minutes │ Servings: 2

Ingredients:

Green beans, whole, frozen - 8 oz of mushrooms, chopped - 1 cup.

Yellow onion, chopped - ¼ cup.

Clove of garlic, minced - 1

Greek yogurt, plain, low fat - ½ cup

Sour cream, low fat - ¼ cup

Corn starch - ½ tsp

Stevia - ¼ pkt Pepper - ½ tsp
Salt - ¼ tsp
Cheddar cheese, low fat, grated - ¼ cup
Grated Parmesan - 1 tbsp
Cooking spray - just enough

Indications:
Wash the vegetables and drain them properly.
Preheat the air fryer to 180 ° C.
Air-fry the beans for 10 minutes, stirring intermittently.
Remove it in a bowl after air frying.
Place the mushrooms, garlic, onion in the frying basket and drizzle with cooking oil to coat.
Air fry for 7 minutes.
Transfer the mixture also to the bowl held with the refried beans in the air.
In a small bowl, mix the sour cream, Greek yogurt, salt, pepper, stevia, and cornstarch.
Transfer the mixture to the bowl of fried vegetables and mix to mix well.

Add the grated cheddar cheese and mix.
Line an oven bowl suitable for the deep fryer and sprinkle some cooking oil.
Transfer the veggie mix into it.
Garnish with grated Parmesan and bake for 30 minutes until the top turns brown.
Serve hot.

Nutritional values per serving:
Calories: 182 | Fat: 6.9 g | Cholesterol: 25 mg | Sodium: 562 mg | Carbohydrates: 19 g | Protein: 14 g

Conclusion

The Optavia diet may be the right choice for you if you focus on the system and thus need to lose weight soon. It will undoubtedly help you shed pounds with its relatively low calorie meal plans; however, it is debatable whether the weight reduction will last if the diet is interrupted.

Before starting any meal replacement plan, carefully analyze if you can implement it, evaluate how much money you can spend, and evaluate how relaxed you are with the level of hunger and disruption in your social life.

When you plan to rely on Optavia to excel in your short-term weight reduction goals, be sure to educate yourself on the healthiest food to keep weight off for an extended period. Often, keep in mind that a low calorie diet is not the best way to lose weight. Talk to your doctor or registered dietitian about the practical improvements you should make to help you reach your goals and build a more satisfying and balanced eating plan.

CPSIA information can be obtained
at www.ICGtesting.com
Printed in the USA
LVHW042205121222
735105LV00044B/2925

9 781803 615158